A REVIEW OF THE RADIOLOGICAL ASSESSMENTS CORPORATION'S FERNALD DOSE RECONSTRUCTION REPORT

Committee on an Assessment of CDC Radiation Studies
Board on Radiation Effects Research
Commission on Life Sciences
National Research Council

NATIONAL ACADEMY PRESS
Washington, DC 1997

NATIONAL ACADEMY PRESS 2101 CONSTITUTION AVENUE, NW, WASHINGTON, D.C. 20418

The project that is the subject of this report was approved by the Governing Board of the National Research Council, whose members are drawn from the councils of the National Academy of Sciences, the National Academy of Engineering, and the Institute of Medicine. The members of the committee responsible for the report were chosen for their special competences and with regard to appropriate balance.

This report has been reviewed by a group other than the authors according to procedures approved by a Report Review Committee consisting of members of the National Academy of Sciences, the National Academy of Engineering, and the Institute of Medicine.

This report was prepared under contract 200-95-0965 between the National Academy of Sciences and the Centers for Disease Control and Prevention.

International Standard Book Number 0-309-05677-2

Additional copies of this report are available from

National Research Council
Board on Radiation Effects Research
Room 342
2101 Constitution Avenue, NW
Washington, D.C. 20418
202 334-2232

Printed in the United States of America

COMMITTEE ON AN ASSESSMENT OF CDC RADIATION STUDIES

WILLIAM J. SCHULL (*Chairman*), University of Texas Health Science Center, Houston, Texas

STEPHAN A. BENJAMIN, Colorado State University, Fort Collins, Colorado

ANDRÉ BOUVILLE, National Cancer Institute, Bethesda, Maryland

PATRICIA A.H. BUFFLER, University of California, Berkeley, California

GEOFFREY G. EICHHOLZ, Georgia Institute of Technology, Atlanta, Georgia

J. CHARLES JENNETT, Texas A&M International University, Laredo, Texas

LEEKA I. KHEIFETS, Electric Power Research Institute, Palo Alto, California

JAMES E. MARTIN, University of Michigan, Ann Arbor, Michigan

CHRISTOPHER B. NELSON, US Environmental Protection Agency, Washington, DC

HENRY D. ROYAL, Mallinckrodt Institute of Radiology, St. Louis, Missouri

ROY E. SHORE, New York University Medical Center, New York, New York

ROBERG G. THOMAS, Bigfork, Montana

HENRY N. WAGNER JR., The Johns Hopkins Medical Institutes, Baltimore, Maryland

JAMES M. WALL, The Christian Century, Chicago, Illinois

NATIONAL RESEARCH COUNCIL STAFF

EVAN B. DOUPLE, Study Director
JOHN D. ZIMBRICK, Director, Board on Radiation Effects Research
DORIS E. TAYLOR, Staff Assistant
NORMAN GROSSBLATT, Editor

SPONSOR'S PROJECT OFFICER

JAMES M. SMITH, Centers for Disease Control and Prevention, Atlanta, Georgia

BOARD ON RADIATION EFFECTS RESEARCH

COMMISSION ON LIFE SCIENCES

THOMAS D. POLLARD (*Chairman*), Salk Institute for Biological Studies, La Jolla, California

FREDERICK R. ANDERSON, Cadwalader, Wickersham & Taft, Washington, DC

JOHN C. BAILAR III, University of Chicago, Illinois

PAUL BERG, Stanford University, Stanford, California

JOHN E. BURRIS, Marine Biological Laboratory, Woods Hole, Massachusetts

SHARON L. DUNWOODY, University of Wisconsin, Madison, Wisconsin California, Riverside, California

GLENN A. CROSBY, Washington State University, Pullman, Washington

URSULA W. GOODENOUGH, Washington University, St. Louis, Missouri

HENRY W. HEIKKINEN, University of Northern Colorado, Greeley, Colorado

HANS J. KENDE, Michican State University, East Lansing, Michigan

SUSAN E. LEEMAN, Boston University School of Medicine, Boston, Massachusetts

THOMAS E. LOVEJOY, Smithsonian Institution, Washington, DC

DONALD R. MATTISON, Graduate School of Public Health, University of Pittsburgh, Pittsburgh, Pennsylvania

JOSEPH E. MURRAY, Wellesley Hills, Massachusetts

EDWARD E. PENHOET, Chiron Corporation, Emeryville, California

EMIL A. PFITZER, Research Institute for Fragrance Materials, Inc., Hackensack, New Jersey

MALCOLM C. PIKE, Norris/USC Comprehensive Cancer Center, Los Angeles, California

HENRY C. PITOT III, McArdle Laboratory for Cancer Research, University of Wisconsin, Madison, Wisconsin

JONATHAN M. SAMET, The Johns Hopkins University, Baltimore, Maryland

CHARLES F. STEVENS, The Salk Institute for Biological Studies, La Jolla, California

JOHN L. VANDEBERG, Southwest Foundation for Biomedical Research, San Antonio, Texas

NATIONAL RESEARCH COUNCIL STAFF

PAUL GILMAN, Executive Director
ALVIN L. LAZEN, Associate Executive Director
SOLVEIG M. PADILLA, Administrative Assistant

The National Academy of Sciences is a private, nonprofit, self-perpetuating society of distinguished scholars engaged in scientific and engineering research, dedicated to the furtherance of science and technology and to their use for the general welfare. Upon the authority of the charter granted to it by the Congress in 1863, the Academy has a mandate that requires it to advise the federal government on scientific and technical matters. Dr. Bruce M. Alberts is president of the National Academy of Sciences.

The National Academy of Engineering was established in 1964, under the charter of the National Academy of Sciences, as a parallel organization of outstanding engineers. It is autonomous in its administration and in the selection of its members, sharing with the National Academy of Sciences the responsibility for advising the federal government. The National Academy of Engineering also sponsors engineering programs aimed at meeting national needs, encourages education and research, and recognizes the superior achievements of engineers. Dr. William A. Wulf is interim president of the National Academy of Engineering.

The Institute of Medicine was established in 1970 by the National Academy of Sciences to secure the services of eminent members of appropriate professions in the examination of policy matters pertaining to the health of the public. The Institute acts under the responsibility given to the National Academy of Sciences by its congressional charter to be an adviser to the federal government and, upon its own initiative, to identify issues of medical care, research, and education. Dr. Kenneth I. Shine is president of the Institute.

The National Research Council was organized by the National Academy of Sciences in 1916 to associate the broad community of science and technology with the Academy's purposes of furthering knowledge and advising the federal government. Functioning in accordance with general policies determined by the Academy, the Council has become the principal operating agency of both the National Academy of Sciences and the National Academy of Engineering in providing services to the government, the public, and the scientific and engineering communities. The Council is administered jointly by both Academies and the Institute of Medicine. Dr. Bruce M. Alberts and Dr. William A. Wulf are chairman and interim vice chairman, respectively, of the National Research Council.

PREFACE

The first specific task requested by the Centers for Disease Control and Prevention (CDC) of the National Research Council's Committee on an Assessment of CDC Radiation Studies was a review of draft reports prepared by the Radiological Assessments Corporation (RAC) pertaining to its efforts to reconstruct environmental doses of radionuclides in the vicinity of the Fernald, Ohio, nuclear facility, the Feed Materials Production Center (FMPC). The facility, some 15 miles northwest of Cincinnati, began operation in 1951 and continued production activities through 1988. (It is now called the Fernald Environmental Management Project, or FEMP.) FMPC converted uranium feed materials (uranium concentrates, uranium compounds recycled from various stages of nuclear-weapons production, and some uranium ores) to uranium metal ingots for machining or extrusion in tubular form. Although uranium processing was the primary activity at FMPC, smaller amounts of thorium were processed intermittently during the middle 1950s and in 1964-1980, and some recycled uranium feed materials were processed beginning in late 1963. These activities and the storage of waste production materials containing radionuclides in silos at the facility led to the release of substantial amounts of uranium dust and radon gas into the environment. The releases raised the possibility of detrimental health effects in people living in the vicinity of the facility.

The primary purpose of RAC's Fernald Dose-Reconstruction Project was to estimate the radiation doses received by members of the public who lived near FMPC between 1950 and 1989. RAC approached its charge through a series of 6 tasks: (1) identifying the release points on the Fernald site; (2) developing the source terms, that is, the quantity, chemical and physical form, and time course of contaminants released to the environment from the facility; (3) identifying the uncertainties or level of confidence in the assessment of the source term; (4) developing environmental transport and dose calculations; (5) identifying and compiling environmental and other data to verify the transport and dose calculations; and (6) presenting the final doses and health risks with their attending uncertainties. Each task culminated in an interim report that was reviewed by the committee. The first interim reports to be reviewed were on radionuclide source terms (task 2) and uncertainties (task 3) for 1960-1962; the committee's review, *Dose*

Reconstruction for the Fernald Nuclear Facility, was published in 1992. Next, the committee was asked to review the report of task 4, to develop methods that could be used to translate the release estimates into concentrations of radioactive materials in the residential environment. The committee's review of those methods, *Dose Reconstruction for the Fernald Nuclear Facility: A Review of Task 4*, was published in 1994. In 1995, the committee submitted a letter report to CDC in response to a request for advice on the methods and future directions of the Fernald project and on their appropriateness and scientific soundness. In that letter, the committee reported its findings and commented on 6 issues for which CDC requested further clarification. The committee endorsed the overall approach being used by RAC in the dose-reconstruction project, judged that the project was generally headed in the right direction, and commended RAC for its thoroughness in addressing all issues carefully, soundly, and persuasively.

RAC's draft report, *Task 6: Radiation Doses and Risk to Residents from FMPC Operations from 1951-1988*, was released in 2 volumes on August 22, 1996. Volume I summarizes the major releases of radionuclides, including releases to the atmosphere, surface water, and groundwater; discusses transport of radionuclides in air and in water; compares environmental measurements with predictions; and estimates the doses received by the public from FMPC releases, the health effects of the estimated doses, and the lifetime risks of cancer associated with each of 9 exposure scenarios. Volume II sets forth in technical detail the methods used in assessing doses and includes 20 appendixes that provide information on the data that were used, the analytic models and methods, and the assumptions inherent in the computations. The present report consists of the committee's review and assessment of those volumes.

The committee members wish to thank the members of the RAC team who briefed the committee on the contents of the reports and answered questions regarding the approaches and methods used in the study. Specifically, RAC president John E. Till and contributing authors Susan K. Rope, Duane W. Schmidt, and Warren K. Sinclair made presentations to the committee. The committee members also wish to express thanks to Doris E. Taylor for her assistance in the preparation of this report and for her administrative assistance.

William J. Schull

Chairman

CONTENTS

EXECUTIVE SUMMARY

A National Research Council Committee on an Assessment of CDC Radiation Studies was asked by the Centers for Disease Control and Prevention to review the final results of the Fernald Dose Reconstruction Project. The purpose of that dose-reconstruction project conducted by Radiological Assessments Corporation (RAC) was to provide to members of the public scientifically sound radiation-dose estimates resulting from the operations of the Feed Materials Production Center (FMPC) at Fernald, Ohio, from 1951 through 1988. Dose reconstruction was necessary because the radiation doses had not been directly measured. The most-accurate method for measuring the doses would have been to measure periodically the uranium or other radionuclides in the bodies of members of the public and to measure the radon in their homes, schools, and places of work. However, direct public dose monitoring was not done at Fernald, for a variety of reasons, including the assumption that a monitoring system would have been intrusive, impractical, expensive, and unnecessary.

To protect the health of the public, an alternative approach, environmental monitoring, has been routinely used. If the radionuclides in the environment are measured and kept below a predefined limit, excessive doses to members of the public can be avoided. That approach has been generally successful, and the risk associated with additional radiation exposure of members of the public has in many cases been smaller than risks associated with large industrial facilities in their vicinities. However, to gain perspective on risks, concerned members of the public have raised questions about what their actual radiation exposures were. How does one know what the doses were if they were not measured? How does one know that all the facts have been disclosed? A limited answer to such questions can be provided by a scientific dose reconstruction that is based on analyses of radionuclide-release data and modeling of exposures of typical members of the public. RAC's final report reviewed in this document represents such a study for the FMPC.

By using dose reconstruction, it is possible to fill some of the gaps in the data. When environmental-monitoring data do not exist, likely values can be reconstructed on the basis of measurements obtained elsewhere under similar conditions or at different times in the same general area. How various radionuclides move through the environment can be estimated by using complex mathematical models that attempt to account for many important physical and chemical properties of the radionuclides. Ultimately, actual or potential doses to people can be approximated with these models and others that estimate how much and for how long the released radionuclides come into contact with members of the public in a given setting.

How good are the dose estimates? Whether the dose estimates are scientifically credible depends on the methods used and the care with which they were used. But even when the best methods are used carefully, dose estimates can be flawed. Gaps in the historical records lead to uncertainty. Occasionally, the gaps can be accurately filled because there is a clear relationship between missing and known data; more often, the relationship between missing and known data is complicated, and assumptions must be made. Such assumptions are necessarily imperfect and add uncertainty to the estimates of dose. Uncertainty is generally expressed not only by stating the best estimate of the dose but also by including a range of possible values. Scientists must acknowledge that uncertainty exists and try to estimate it. But it can be reduced only if more-relevant data are available. Even estimating the amount of uncertainty is subject to uncertainty. As with the dose estimates themselves, whether the uncertainty estimates are scientifically sound depends on the methods used and the care with which they are applied.

This committee concludes that the methods used in the Fernald Dose Reconstruction Project are appropriate and scientifically sound—indeed, often innovative. The uncertainty in the final dose estimates results mainly from gaps in the environmental-monitoring record and from the assumptions that are required to go from the reasonably well-known amounts of radionuclides released (the source term) to descriptions of how they were transported through the environment, potentially exposing members of the public. Added to those are the uncertainties in the cancer-risk coefficients that have been applied. Given the extensive record search, it is unlikely that important documents that would reduce the uncertainty or change the magnitude of the dose estimates remain to be discovered.

There are some differences between the approaches used by RAC and approaches that might have been recommended by the National Research Council committee. Those differences are to be expected when complex tasks such as dose reconstruction are undertaken and there are significant gaps in the historic record. In the opinion of the committee, the RAC approach has resulted in an overestimation of doses to people from exposure to radon. This overestimation of the doses from radon is discussed in detail in the body of the present report.

The RAC dose reconstruction work reviewed by this committee was carefully done and covered all known pathways of exposure of the surrounding population. The committee is concerned that RAC's overestimation of doses received by the population from radon, although prudent, might produce some undeserved apprehension on the part of some citizens and should be carefully presented. While parts of the summary booklet of the report intended to present the risk estimations are well written, other parts do a poor job of overall risk communication. In particular, certain figures are misleading and should be revised. The committee recommends that RAC present separate estimates for some of the risk scenarios contingent on whether the person is a smoker or nonsmoker. In addition, the committee believes that the RAC report underestimates the uncertainties associated with its risk estimates. Although it is difficult to estimate the precise extent of overestimation, it might be a factor of 4 or 6 and needs to be corrected. The above issues might be important factors if CDC decides to evaluate whether an epidemiologic study of the exposed population should be proposed.

INTRODUCTION

Under a memorandum of understanding concluded with the US Department of Energy (DOE) in December 1990, the US Department of Health and Human Services, through its Centers for Disease Control and Prevention (CDC), has been conducting a series of studies to assess the possible health consequences of exposure to releases of radioactive materials from DOE-managed nuclear facilities throughout the United States. In recent years, persons living around those facilities have become increasingly concerned that radioactive materials emanating from the facilities have affected their health. At CDC's request, the Board on Radiation Effects Research in the National Research Council (NRC) Commission on Life Sciences organized the Committee on an Assessment of CDC Radiation Studies to provide scientific advice to CDC's Center for Environmental Health and Injury Control and to evaluate the quality and completeness of CDC's assessments.

The NRC committee's charge is as follows:

- To review and comment on the design, methods, analysis, statistical reliability, and scientific interpretation of dose-reconstruction studies and related epidemiologic followup studies.
- To recommend ways to strengthen study protocols and analyses so that the scientific validity of the study results can be ensured.

The first specific task requested by CDC was a review of draft reports prepared by the Radiological Assessments Corporation (RAC) pertaining to its efforts to reconstruct environmental doses due to releases of radionuclides in the vicinity of the Fernald, Ohio, nuclear facility, the Feed Materials Production Center (FMPC). FMPC, some 15 miles to the northwest of Cincinnati, began operation in 1951 and continued production activities until 1988. FMPC converted uranium feed materials (uranium concentrates, uranium compounds recycled from various stages of nuclear-weapons production, and some uranium ores) to uranium metal ingots for machining or extrusion in tubular form. Although uranium processing was the primary activity at FMPC, smaller amounts of thorium were processed intermittently during the middle 1950s and in 1964-1980, and some recycled uranium feed materials were processed beginning in late 1963. These activities and the storage of waste production materials containing radionuclides in silos at the facility led to the release of substantial amounts of uranium dust and radon gas into the environment. The releases raised the possibility of detrimental health effects in people living in the vicinity of the facility. It was that possibility that RAC was charged with assessing.

RAC approached its charge through a series of 6 tasks: (1) identifying the release points on the Fernald site; (2) developing the source terms, that is, the quantity, chemical and physical form, and time course of contaminants released to the environment from the facility; (3) identifying the uncertainties or level of confidence in the assessment of the source terms; (4) developing environmental transport and dose calculations; (5) identifying and compiling environmental and other data to verify the transport and dose calculations; and (6) presenting the final doses and health risks with their attending uncertainties. Each task culminated in an interim report that was reviewed by the committee. Consequently, there has been some feedback between the committee and RAC in the course of this work as the committee communicated some of its concerns in the earlier stages.

The first RAC drafts reported on by the Research Council committee covered the period 1960-1962 and dealt with radionuclide source terms (task 2) and uncertainties (task 3); the committee's review, *Dose Reconstruction for the Fernald Nuclear Facility*, was published in 1992 (NRC 1992). Next, the committee was asked to review the report of task 4, to develop methods that could be used to translate the release estimates into concentrations of radioactive materials in the residential environment. The committee's review of those methods, *Dose Reconstruction for the Fernald Nuclear Facility: A Review of Task 4*, was published in 1994 (NRC 1994). In 1995, the committee submitted a letter report to CDC in response to a request for advice on the methods and future directions of the Fernald project and on their appropriateness and scientific soundness. In that letter, the committee reported its findings and commented on 6 issues for which CDC requested further clarification. The committee endorsed the overall approach being used by RAC in the dose-reconstruction project, judged that the project was generally headed in the right direction, and commended RAC for its thoroughness in addressing all issues carefully, soundly, and persuasively.

On August 1-2, 1996, at the National Academy of Sciences Beckman Center in Irvine, California, the committee was briefed by John Till and members of the RAC staff on the methods used for task 6; however, no information was presented on the dose estimates themselves. RAC's draft report, *Task 6: Radiation Doses and Risk to Residents from FMPC Operations from 1951-1988*, was released in 2 volumes on August 22, 1996. Volume I, summarizes the major releases of radionuclides, including releases to the atmosphere, surface water, and groundwater; discusses transport of radionuclides in air and in water; compares environmental measurements with predictions, and estimates the doses received by the public from FMPC releases, the health effects of the estimated doses, and the lifetime risk of cancer associated with each of 9 exposure scenarios. Volume II sets forth in technical detail the methods used in assessing doses and includes 20 appendixes that provide information on the data that were used, the analytic models and methods, and the assumptions inherent in the computations. A second briefing was held on September 19-20, 1996, in Washington, DC, after the public release of the report; on this occasion the committee completed its review of the task 6 draft documents, including a third document, a summary addressed to the lay audience. The present committee report consists of the committee's review and assessment of those 3 documents.

ENVIRONMENTAL RELEASES

Environmental radionuclide releases can lead to the contamination of air, soil, surface water and groundwater. Each of those pathways must be evaluated if the health consequences of releases are to be reliably assessed. Of primary concern at FMPC are the releases of uranium and radon.

Uranium

The RAC report offers 310,000 kg as the best estimate of the release of uranium to the atmosphere over the period of operation of the FMPC. This estimate is based on data from dust collectors, plants 2 and 3, plant 8 scrubbers, and miscellaneous other sources. That release to the atmosphere is substantially larger than uranium releases in liquid effluents and the releases of thorium and other radionuclides. Moreover, the atmospheric uranium releases are of greater importance because the material is more available for exposure of off site populations. Particle-size analysis is important in terms of eventual radiation dose calculations for the lung since particles of certain sizes are quickly propelled out of the pulmonary tree, swallowed, and no longer available to expose the lung.

Overall, the uranium-release estimates are well done and reflect the committee's earlier comments on the source-term modeling. However, the sums of the median quantities in tables 2-5 are inconsistent, and the total is closer to 290,000 than to 310,000 kg.

Radon

Radon released from the waste stored in the K-65 silos, which were partially sunk below ground level, constitutes the principal source of radiation exposure off site, so it is important to estimate it as reliably as possible. The RAC team has chosen to derive its source term from 1986 gamma-ray measurements of the radon accumulated under the silo dome. The release of radon from this source to the environment is assumed to have been unlimited and driven by thermal pumping before the dome was sealed in 1979 and by diffusion through cracks in the dome since then. Only one measurement of radon concentration in the head space, made in 1987, has been reported to provide direct confirmation of the radon concentration (see figure 14 in volume I of the RAC report). The model derived from the gamma-ray measurements has been referred to by RAC as the "preferred method."

The committee has proposed the use of what has been termed the "conventional method" both to simplify assumptions and to validate the assumed source term by deriving the radon inventory in the head space from the reported radium inventory in the waste mass. The detailed calculation involved is outlined in the appendix "Additional Comments," beginning on page 36 of the present report. The main result of the conventional method is to indicate a substantially lower radon release rate than was obtained with the RAC's preferred method, based on the principle that radon cannot be released from the dome faster than it emanates from the waste mass. The lower release rate is consistent with the few available air measurements off site which are below the concentrations predicted with the preferred method.

The practical implications of the conventional method are to lower the amount of radon released by a factor of 2-3 and increase the range of uncertainties by a factor of 2 or 3. A qualitative assessment of the input data and parameters used in the preferred method indicates that the uncertainty depicted in figure 17 of volume I of the RAC report is unrealistically small and should be increased substantially. In contrast, figure 17 assigns too large an uncertainty to the conventional method, in the committee's view.

It should be noted that the releases estimated by RAC are larger than the Mound Laboratory measurements as shown in figure N-3 of volume II. Those estimates suggest that the stated radium inventories in the K-65 silo residues are too low and the estimated release rates are too high. The only available measurements, at the crosswind station BS-6, while validating the model in the usual sense, also seem to support a much lower release rate than estimated. Overall, the suggested release rates of about 6,200 Ci/yr before 1979 and about 950 Ci/yr for 1980-1987 seem to be grossly overestimated. Such estimation would result in an overestimate of the radon-progeny exposure of off site populations.

TRANSPORT IN THE ENVIRONMENT

Doses to real or hypothetical people hinge not only on the magnitude of a source, but also on how the radionuclides released are transported in the environment. Transport varies with the nuclide and the medium through which transport occurs, that is, surface water, groundwater, or soil. Primary sources of exposure assignable to the Fernald facility are uranium dust and radon gas and its progeny.

Uranium

In 1994, the committee reviewed a draft report of task 4 of the Fernald Dosimetry Reconstruction Project, *Environmental Pathways—Models and Validation*. Most of the committee's comments (NRC 1994) have been taken into account, but some seem to have been disregarded.

The GARDEN model, which deals with the intake of radionuclides via ingestion, seems not to have included the contamination of fresh fruit and bakery products, which, according to National Council on Radiation Protection and Measurements report 77 (NCRP 1984), are among the 5 food categories that contribute the most to intake of background uranium in the United States. The GARDEN model also estimates radionuclide concentrations of raw agricultural products, but people consume food after some handling and preparation, such as washing and removal of the outer leaves of green vegetables, peeling and cooking of potatoes, and cooking of meat products. The report does not discuss the methods or parameter values needed to estimate radionuclide concentrations of prepared foodstuffs.

It is not clear how the soluble and insoluble forms of uranium are characterized and treated in the environmental-transport model. In volume II, appendix C, it is assumed that 35% of the uranium deposited on the ground is in a soluble form that migrates rapidly through the upper layer of soil. Presumably, the soluble and insoluble fractions of uranium will lead to widely different concentrations in some foodstuffs.

Large amounts of pulverized uranium were released from several buildings during the early years, as shown in the RAC report in table 5 of volume I, for a total of about 276,000 kg in elemental or oxide form. Most of this material was relatively coarse or associated with mist droplets (see figure 24), settled close to the point of release, and might have been removed in surface runoff. The meteorologic model described seems to account adequately for the fraction of this airborne release that moved beyond the fence line (see figure 22). The other uranium releases to the environment were contained in liquid effluents consisting of 3 components: monitored plant drain discharges to the Great Miami River; surface runoff, mainly to Paddy's Run Creek; and soil seepage followed by leakage into the subsurface aquifer. In general, these pathways have been treated adequately in the report. The only exception is the assumed seepage of uranium into the subsurface aquifer from Paddy's Run. To the committee, that does not seem to be a credible pathway. Vertical migration of uranium from contaminated soil into the aquifer seems to be a more credible pathway to give rise to the slowly moving groundwater plume described in figure F-1.

The committee has questioned the particle size distribution of the airborne uranium particles given in the report because it affects the transport characteristics and the predicted health effects of inhalation. However, in the overall perspective, any divergences in the assumed size distribution are probably of only secondary importance, and the committee accepts the uranium transport estimates as they stand.

Radon and Its Progeny

Radon is a noble gas, and its dispersion in the atmosphere is governed by a simple diffusion model, as described in the report. However, any biologic effects are due to the decay products of the disintegration of radon into a series of short-lived polonium, bismuth, and lead isotopes, collectively referred to as radon progeny. These isotopes rapidly attach themselves to aerosol particles in the atmosphere, and both transport characteristics and inhalation dynamics are affected by the proportion of attached and unattached radon-progeny atoms. The model assumes equal atmospheric transport for both categories, which might be reasonable under the circumstances. However, plant operations before 1970 undoubtedly resulted in a dustier atmosphere with a higher attachment ratio, and a proportion attached to coarser particles was removed rapidly, on site, by local fallout. Indoor exposure off site resulted almost entirely from radon transport alone.

MODEL VALIDATION

The retrospective assessment of doses and risks necessarily involves the interplay of observations or measurements at specific times or locations and a construct of the events that presumably underlie the observations. This construct, or model, is used to predict what happened at times or locations for which direct observations are not available or are inadequate to provide reasonable assurance that observed values are appropriate. Various potentially applicable models can be envisaged a priori in any given situation, but the choice of the appropriate one centers on accuracy and precision in predicting measured values and hence, presumably, values that are necessary but not available. Testing of such reliability is known as model validation, and it is central to all reconstructions. In the end, model validation requires a comparison of predicted values with independent measured values, within the limits of uncertainty for both. Well-established measurements are often referred to as "benchmarks." In the present case, few relevant measurements were available for either the airborne or the liquid pathways, and the extent of model validation can be considered only qualitative.

Uranium, thorium, radium, plutonium, neptunium, cesium, ruthenium, technetium, and strontium radionuclides were all supposedly considered in the mathematical model describing transport of these radionuclides into groundwater, air, and soil (for example, see table 11 of the RAC report for groundwater). However, none of the fission products were actually followed in any detail after a screening assessment showed them to be of minor consequence. Multiple site-specific receptor locations were examined, and the examination considered the multiple release points within the FMPC production area, the physical and chemical characteristics of the release sources, the rate of diffusion as a function of the distance between the site-specific receptor locations and the multiple release points, the size distribution of the wet and dry particles, the resuspension into air of material previously deposited on the ground, the runoff and leaching of material deposited on soil, the rate of radioactive decay, and the biologic pathways through exposed persons. The atmospheric-dispersion models used to estimate ground-level air concentration at specific locations incorporated local meteorologic data available after August 1986, when a meteorologic tower began full operation. To account for the meteorologic conditions during the years before 1987, 4 types of approximations were used to provide information about wind conditions during the period from the beginning of operation of the plant until 1987. It was concluded that the observed data from the meteorologic tower after August 1986 were the most representative of all those before 1987. The mean wind speed at the Cincinnati airport was not considered reliable for use in the model because direct comparison indicated mean wind speeds frequently twice as high as the measurements made at FMPC.

The short period for which actual meteorologic records were made is a severe limitation. Nevertheless, the comparisons of other sites and the use of simulated environmental conditions afford a degree of confidence that there are no large errors in the meteorologic data or in the atmospheric-dispersion models used.

To compare model-predicted and observed concentrations of uranium, the differences between the 2 values at each of multiple sites were expressed as a predicted:observed (P/O) ratio, where

$$\text{geometric bias (all sites)} = \exp\left[\Sigma \ln (P_i/O_i)/n\right],$$

in which the summation is across all times and sites and P_i is the predicted concentration at the location at time i, O_i is the observed concentration, and n is the number of locations or times.

Whenever parameter values are estimates rather than measurements, the use of mathematical models leads to larger uncertainty in the calculated results. Such uncertainty also results from errors in observed measurements and in the extrapolation from measurements to predictions of missing measurements. Uncertainty is expressed by calculating the range of releases, doses, or risks of health effects. The results have been expressed as the 5th to 95th percentiles; that is, 90% of RAC's predicted values fall within these limits. The 5th and 95th percentiles describing the release of uranium span a range of a factor of 5 in the estimates in the case of soil deposition of uranium. For example, on page C-8 of volume II, the releases are 720,000 kg (95%) and 130,000 kg (5%), a factor of 5-6. That was also the case with respect to uncertainty in the estimation of airborne releases of uranium. For another example, the validation results for uranium were as follows (table 17):

	Time	Geometric bias	Uncertainty in bias
Air (perimeter)	1958-1971	1.0	0.6-1.8
Air (boundary)	1972-1988	1.0	0.6-1.6
Gummed film	1954-1964	0.4	0.3-0.7
Soil	1959, 1971-1988	1.1	0.7-1.7

Modeling the deposition of uranium on the ground was more difficult than modeling air concentrations. Observations based on gummed-film monitoring were compared with predicted values. Deposition predicted for 1954-1956 was in poor agreement with observations, but deposition predicted for 1957-1964 was in better agreement with observations made at that time.

It was possible to compare measurements of uranium in the soil and water with those predicted by the mathematical models, which of necessity included best estimates and approximations of parameters in the model. The release estimates were based, for example, on production information. An example of validation is the comparison of the uranium air-monitoring results from 1986-1988 with the concentrations predicted by the model. Most of the environmental monitoring from which data are available for the early days of the operation of the plant involved only uranium.

Differences between the recent calculations and those reported in 1986 by Stevenson and Hardy were adequately addressed and can be accounted for by the differences in the conditions examined, for example, the depth of soil that was considered. Stevenson and Hardy (1986) considered the top 5 cm of soil, whereas RAC considered the top 10 cm.

Measurements of radon at boundary monitoring stations before and after the silo domes were sealed were proportional to predicted decreases based on the model (see page 69 of the RAC report). Unfortunately, few observation data were available for validation of the release of radon from the silos during the periods of highest releases. From 1980 until the present, the observed radon concentrations in air at multiple boundary air-monitoring stations were similar to those calculated with the radon-dispersion model. For 1986-1991, hourly measurements of radon in air agreed well with predicted large fluctuations related to time of day.

A recapitulation of uncertainties is given in volume II figure M-9, covering both uranium and radon concentrations in air. Well-known statistical methods, some of recent origin, were used in the assessments. For example, Gaussian plume-dispersion models, representation of uncertainties with probability distributions, and Monte Carlo techniques were used.

In general, for both uranium and radon in soil, air, and water, the agreement between predicted and observed concentrations was acceptable. RAC's overall uncertainty in the validation of the releases was a factor of about 5.

DOSE ESTIMATES

Doses to the public from FMPC releases were assessed through atmospheric, surface-water, and groundwater pathways. All important determinants of the dose received were included: the distance and direction of a person's residence and work location in relation to the center of the facility; the time of day and duration that the person spent in the area; the time spent indoors and associated breathing rates and air-turnover; the time spent outdoors and associated breathing rates; the use of contaminated water for drinking, irrigation, and swimming; and the ingestion of contaminated foodstuffs and soil. Those characteristics were allowed to vary for several periods and individual lifestyles (from preschool to employment). However, the RAC authors do not clearly present which parameters are most influential in determining dose, nor do they present the range or distribution of doses to the public from the FMPC releases. Rather, they develop 9 scenarios to represent people born from 1946 to 1970 who lived continuously in the 10-km area around the facility. These scenarios were presented as representative, but the doses presented were biased to the higher end by the focus on people born during the early operation of the facility (6 of 9 scenarios) and the assumption that people spent all this time in the area under consideration. It is unclear whether people who have lived near FMPC will be able to relate the scenarios to their own experiences. Moreover, given the paucity of information on the importance of various characteristics, it would be impossible for a given person to determine whether the difference between his or her experience and the scenarios might lead to a higher or lower dose.

The main purpose of estimating doses from the radon-decay products in the task 6 draft report is to be able to compare them with doses to the organs and tissues from other sources. The committee makes the following recommendations regarding the dose comparison. First, the methods used to calculate lung doses from radon decay products and from other sources must be consistent for the dose comparison to be meaningful. RAC has calculated the dose to the bronchial epithelium by using an NCRP method (NCRP 1984), but the average lung dose from other inhaled radionuclides is calculated by using the method from ICRP Publication 30 (ICRP 1988). Second, the uncertainties in such estimates should be acknowledged and quantified. In practice, the risk from radon-product exposure is estimated from the radon decay-product exposure, not from a dose estimate. The committee notes that the risk per unit dose for radon decay products in this report has been specifically calculated to be consistent with the risk per unit exposure from the BEIR IV report (NRC 1988) and is different from the risk per unit dose for other radionuclides. The lung doses from radon decay products and uranium in figure 46 of the RAC report are not directly comparable.

Dose reconstruction is necessarily both a retrospective activity and a site-specific one that often requires the reconstruction of events that occurred decades earlier. Reconstruction, depending as it commonly does on incomplete and often imperfect data, has its uncertainties. The sources of uncertainty include the need to estimate critical parameters in the modeling process when data are scarce or not available; the need to extrapolate observations made at one time to other times for which necessary data are absent; the need to assess the reliability of individual-specific information on lifestyle and residence, for example, in translating estimates of health risk from one population to another to which the risks might not be fully applicable; and the need to allow for the approximate nature of mathematical models of complex physical and biologic processes. Identification of those sources of uncertainty and estimation of their possible effects on the results of a dose reconstruction make up what is referred to as uncertainty analysis. The intent of such analysis is to determine the level of confidence that can be placed in the results of the reconstruction itself. Uncertainty analysis provides a measure of the credibility to be assigned to the reconstruction and is an integral part of the reconstruction process.

The RAC report has gone to exceptional lengths to assess and allow for uncertainties in the components that define exposure (uncertainties in the size of the environmental radiation releases and environmental transport). However, uncertainties pertaining to interindividual variation in the intake of radioactive materials were taken into account inadequately. In particular, as previously stated, 9 hypothetical "representative" scenarios pertaining to variations in when and where persons lived and to some lifestyle and dietary habits were defined. The variations were then assumed to define each individual's intake and metabolism of the radionuclides in question *without error* (that is, no uncertainty was attached to these factors). Even if one assumes that a hypothetical individual's lifestyle and dietary factors have no uncertainty because they are "givens" for a particular scenario, uncertainties are still attached to almost all these factors. To name a few, for the factors pertaining to time spent indoors and outdoors, there would be an uncertainty range attached to the "indoor particle factor" (ratio of indoor to outdoor particle concentrations) that would be set at 0.7:1. There would likewise be a distribution of air turnover rates (0.4 h^{-1} assumed) in houses, schools, and so on. In the estimated radionuclide intakes from various classes of foods and water, the assumption is made that absolute intakes were constants for a given age and sex (for example, a 7-year-old girl would eat *x* amount of vegetables per year without variation) and that the radionuclide contamination would be an equivalent constant (for example, for all possible mixes of vegetable types, meat types, or fish types). There would clearly be distributions of radionuclides that would impart uncertainty to the estimates that should have been considered in arriving at overall estimates of uncertainty in doses. Physiologic factors would also contribute uncertainty: variations in breathing rates, lung size, and particle-expulsion efficiency; variations in absorption, metabolism, and retention times of radionuclides; and so on.

Although the RAC report considers only the 9 hypothetical "representative" persons with fixed characteristics, if the doses to the Fernald population are to be modeled realistically, uncertainty estimates have to factor in uncertainties in the assessed or imputed lifestyles and intakes and uncertainties in the dose-conversion factors. For instance, individual reports of the percentage of time spent indoors or the degree of indoor vs. outdoor physical activity might be imprecise, inaccurate, or both.

Intensive studies to validate reported dietary intakes of nutrients have typically reported validity coefficients in the range of only 0.35-0.7 (for example, Willett and others 1985; Rimm and others 1992); that indicates appreciable uncertainty in the assessment of dietary intake.

According to the report (table S-14, page S-25), uncertainties in the estimation of biologic factors involved in estimating risks associated with uranium and thorium include the following:

	5th percentile	95th percentile
Uncertainty in RBE	0.5	1.5
Uncertainty in statistics	0.5	1.5
Other uncertainties	0.5	2
Combined uncertainty	0.33	2.6

The uncertainty due to the above factors alone results in an 8-fold difference between the 5th percentile and the 95th percentile.

In the case of radon (table S-17, page S-27), the range of uncertainties is as follows:

	5th percentile	95th percentile
Statistics	0.59	1.7
Dosimetry	0.71	1.4
Modeling and smoking	0.5	2
Other	0.5	2
Combined	0.33	3.3

As mentioned previously, the committee believes that the imputed range of uncertainty for radon dosimetry, given above, is unrealistically narrow.

A final comment should be made about why the newer respiratory tract model of the International Commission on Radiological Protection (ICRP 1994a) was not used in the RAC report. The principal reason is that at the time of the task 4 report (1993), in which mathematical models were developed to describe the movement of radionuclides released from the site into the environment and to calculate the radiation doses to residents, the new ICRP lung model was not yet available. In the present work, low- and high-linear energy transfer (LET) dose coefficients were developed, as well as age-related differences in the dose coefficients. Radiation-risk programs from the US Environmental Protection Agency (EPA) and ICRP report 30 (ICRP 1988) models were used in adjusting dosimetry for low and high LET. Oak Ridge National Laboratory reports were used to develop age-dependent effects on dose coefficients. Under the circumstances, that is acceptable, and a change in methods would not substantially affect the outcome of this project, given the inherent range of uncertainties.

Although an assessment of the magnitude of the intraindividual and interindividual uncertainties compared with the magnitude of uncertainties in the environmental-release and transport components has to our knowledge not been performed, the committee suspects that the 2 magnitudes are similar. Accordingly, the committee concludes that the magnitude of dose uncertainties is probably substantially underestimated in the RAC report.

HEALTH EFFECTS

Untoward health effects in members of the public residing in the vicinity of FMPC could arise through exposure to ionizing radiation, through the radiations emitted by radionuclides released from the facility, through the chemical toxicity of uranium released from the facility, or from other causes. The possible effects of the releases from the facility are considered in this report.

Radiation-related effects

The primary result of the Fernald Dose Reconstruction Project is an estimate of the probability that the radiation dose received by members of the public during the operation of FMPC might result in cancer, particularly lung cancer. Before the dose-reconstruction project, most scientists believed that the radiation dose to members of the public at Fernald was smaller than that from other sources of radiation exposure (such as radon in homes) and that the radiation dose from inhalation of uranium released into the environment would be the dominant source of the public's radiation exposure. Results of the dose-reconstruction project indicate 2 major points: that the radiation doses resulting from the facility were small relative to background radiation (see tables 22 and 23 in the RAC report) and that radon from the K-65 silos was a more important source of radiation exposure than was inhalation of uranium. The uncertainty of the radon exposures is larger than the uncertainty of the uranium exposures simply because fewer release or environmental data were available on which to base the dose-reconstruction models or to corroborate their predictions.

Most estimates of risk associated with exposure to radon are based on exposure to radon progeny in terms of working-level months (WLM) or in SI units ($Jm^{-3}s$). The methods used by RAC are based on estimating the concentrations of radon progeny where people resided. It would have been straightforward to compute WLM at this point. However, RAC computed the absorbed dose to the bronchial epithelium. Then (see page S-6) they used an inverse conversion from dose back to WLM for comparing risk. This is very unconventional.

There is ample evidence that very high doses of radon cause an increase in lung cancer in humans. Numerous studies in the United States and in other countries have confirmed that uranium miners have a measurable increase in lung cancer that is clearly related to radon exposure. For the purposes of protecting the public from the health effects of radiation exposure, many scientists and public-health officials have assumed that even small doses of radiation (from radon or other sources) cause cancer and that the number of cancers that radiation causes is linearly related to the radiation dose. That is called the linear no-threshold hypothesis. There are large uncertainties in the epidemiologic studies from which the hypothesis and the associated risk coefficients are derived. Obtaining direct evidence as to whether radon or other sources of radiation cause cancer at low doses is difficult for a number of reasons. First, the number of radiation-caused cancers that are predicted by the linear no-threshold hypothesis at low doses is small, compared with the natural incidence of cancer; when the difference is small, it is nearly impossible to detect it unless the exposed population is very large. Second, radiation-caused cancers are indistinguishable from non-radiation-related cancers. Third, most cancers occur long after the exposure to radiation; the determination of a possible cause-effect relationship necessitates, as in the Fernald experience, retrospective estimation of dose over long periods, which leads to large uncertainty in the estimated doses. The more uncertainty there is in the estimates of dose, the more difficult it is to identify potential increases in risk.

Chemical toxicity

The harmful chemical effects of uranium might be larger than the harmful effects of the radiation dose. The RAC report's discussion of the chemical toxicity of uranium is confusing. Unlike cancer, the major end point for radiation effects, the end points for the chemical toxicity of uranium vary from study to study, and the threshold dose for toxic effects depends on the end point that is used. To some extent, the "controversy" about the threshold for the toxic effects of uranium can be explained by the use of different end points in different studies.

Many toxicants (such as alcohol) cause damage that can be detected and can be reversed. The kidney has excess functional capacity, so even permanent damage might not result in clinically important decreases in renal function. On the basis of studies of occupationally exposed uranium workers, it is unlikely that even the most highly exposed members of the public living near Fernald suffered important renal damage from their exposure to chronic or acute releases of uranium.

Uncertainty in the estimation of the health effects

In defining various dose and risk-estimate parameters, the RAC report has leaned in the conservative direction, that is, toward overestimating dose and risk. Although the degree of overestimation varies among different factors, the cumulative effect might be substantial. On the dose-conversion and risk-estimation side, the following factors have led to an overestimate of risk (see also the additional specific comments in the appendix of this report):

- The report assumes that environmental radon produces risk that is larger than that associated with radon among miners, whereas a Research Council report (NRC 1991) indicates a factor of 0.7-0.8 on the basis of differences in breathing rates, fraction unattached to particles, and other conditions.
- RAC incorporated a radon age 0-19 risk factor of 2, whereas a Research Council BEIR IV report (NRC 1988) indicates that a factor of 1 appears appropriate.
- RAC multiplied the all-age risk coefficient (rather than the adult risk coefficient) by 2 for irradiation at ages 0-19.
- RAC incorporated a sex factor larger than 1 (numeric details not given, but only shown on a graph in volume II, page S-11), whereas there is little evidence of a gender difference for the organs that were under consideration.
- Of the several estimates of radon risk available from authoritative bodies, RAC chose the highest (and oldest) estimate available as a starting point.
- The radon risk estimates are unduly high for nonsmokers (whose lifetime radon risk is one-fourth to one-third that for smokers).
- The report overemphasizes the importance of radon-dose estimates. In practice, lung-cancer risk is estimated directly from exposure to radon-decay products (progeny). Such risk estimates are typically about one-third to one-half those based on dose.

A radon dose-conversion factor for general-population exposure relative to miners' exposure (called the K factor) has been given by the Research Council (NRC 1991) as about 0.8 for ages under 10 and 0.7 otherwise. RAC did not apply this factor but claims that "part of this difference is already accounted for in the conversion factor from WLM to rads" (page S-6, line 1); but the relative conversion factor that it refers to (0.65/0.5 = 1.3) appears to be in the opposite direction to the K factor. The discussion of a lung-cancer risk coefficient (see pages S-5 and S-6 in volume II) is incomplete, although the final result appears reasonable. Notably lacking was any discussion of uncertainties in radon risk estimates associated with smoking and with other lung-cancer cofactors (such as silica, arsenic, and diesel exhaust) in the mining studies. As mentioned above, the RAC assessment of lung-cancer risk did not take into account the apparent interaction between radon exposure and smoking. The joint analyses of the miner data have resulted in a larger than additive relation between smoking and radon exposure with respect to lung cancer (Lubin and others 1995). By taking the average risk across both smokers and nonsmokers, RAC has thereby overestimated the lifetime risk for nonsmokers and underestimated it for smokers. In particular, the absolute risks associated with radon for smokers are about 3-4 times higher than those for nonsmokers. Lubin and others (1995) have found relative risks 3 times higher for nonsmokers than smokers, but when the relative risks are applied to the baseline rate among nonsmokers, which is one-tenth that of smokers, the absolute risk is one-fourth to one-third in nonsmokers. Ignoring a difference that large is questionable. It is suggested that RAC present separate estimates for at least the larger risk scenarios contingent on whether the person is a smoker or nonsmoker.

The RAC examined the estimates of lung-cancer risk from uranium-worker studies to compare them with the risk estimate from the highest doses received by atomic-bomb survivors. In comparing the major study of multiple uranium facilities by Dupree and others (1995) (page S-8 in volume II) with other results, RAC did not use the overall risk estimate of Dupree and others, but rather concentrated on an ad hoc subgroup. For combined internal and external radiation dose, Dupree and others (1995) found a relative risk (RR) for total lung dose of 1.000 (95% CI, 0.859-1.094), whereas for internal irradiation alone the RR was 1.009 (CI, 0.983-1.036); neither indicates an increased risk. That was based on generally larger doses than the residents around Fernald received (and, in fact, the study of Dupree and others included the Fernald-worker population), so it should provide a measure of assurance to the residents regarding their exposure to uranium dust. Similarly, the other major multifacility uranium-worker study (Waxweiler and others 1983) could not detect an association between uranium exposure and lung-cancer risk at the doses the workers received.

Referring to the worker studies in volume II page S-8, the report says, "whenever an estimate of risk is possible, the result is not very different from what would be expected on the basis of the A-bomb survivor data." But the authors have selected only subsets of data and findings that support an increased risk, rather than looking at the data as a whole, which suggest that the risk is very small.

The committee is concerned about the presentation of risks on page S-11 and in table S-3 and figure S-1 in volume II. In the Japanese atomic-bomb study (on which the risk estimates are based), much of the excess in lifetime radiation risks for females over that for males comes about by virtue of risks to the female breast and genital organs. There is little evidence for assuming higher female risks for the organs of interest in the present RAC study. In particular, the Research Council's BEIR IV report (NRC 1988) indicates that the lifetime risk of lung cancer associated with radon exposure is equal for males and females.

With respect to age adjustment for radon exposure (as on page S-12), a recent study indicated that there is no evident age differential in risk associated with radon exposure (ICRP 1994b). However, RAC chose to use an age-adjustment factor of 2 for exposures occurring before age 20 and 1 after age 20. It thereby increased the risk estimates appreciably for the various scenarios. The age bias played a major role in that most of the 9 hypothetical scenarios assumed that exposure was primarily in childhood. If RAC wished to maintain the same overall risk coefficient as that used by ICRP or BEIR IV, while maintaining an age factor, it should have made the juvenile factor somewhat larger than 1 but the adult factor somewhat less than 1. Instead, by virtue of the age adjustment, it has arbitrarily projected larger risks than have the studies that used the major data sets. In a similar vein, this section projects a higher risk for females than for males. In contrast, the Research Council's BEIR IV report (page 48) states that "the committee could identify no biologic rationale for considering that sex influences the development of radon-related carcinoma of the lung. . . . The relative risks appear to be similar in males and females when quantitative aspects of smoking habits are adjusted for."

With respect to the uncertainties in risk estimation, although the discussion covers the principal categories of uncertainty, a closer inspection of the categories shows that not all sources of uncertainty are covered within the categories. For example, RAC mentions that they do not include uncertainties in some parameter values, such as dose conversion factors (page S-24).

It is difficult even for scientists to understand the nuances of a 90% uncertainty range so as to interpret it appropriately. Hence, it would be helpful in the summary booklet to have a paragraph describing it. One common misconception about uncertainty ranges is that all possible values in the range are equally likely. It would therefore be informative to state the concept that values near the median or mean are appreciably more likely than ones out on the tails and to illustrate it with a sample probability-distribution curve from one of the Monte Carlo simulations superimposed on error bars. The last paragraph on page S-31 would be better balanced (and less alarming to the public) if RAC had also described how small the risks might be (at the 5th percentile), rather than emphasizing only the 95th-percentile risk.

Several figures in the RAC report are confusing or misleading. For example, the legend to figure 48 on page 88 of volume I indicates that cumulative doses are being presented and presumably all contributions are being added together. It is not clear why the 5% quantile always corresponds exactly to background—does this mean that the central 90% interval of the excess dose from Fernald is simply stacked on top of the background? It is not clear how the median in scenario 5 can be below the contribution of background if they are added together. Figure 51 is another example where the graph is misleading. Why is there no uncertainty associated with background? Box plots might be a more appropriate method for comparing central tendencies, spreads, and tails in a simple and consistent manner. Side-by-side bar graphs similar to figure 46 would also illustrate the comparison that is intended and would eliminate much of the confusion.

The public would probably like a means to compare the risk from the silo radon emanations with the levels of exposure that are common to the general public. To provide a context for the radon doses from the silos, RAC compares them with the background radon dose in homes for the same number of years (see table 23 on page 86 and the discussion on page 87 in volume I). A more useful comparison would probably be with the background radon dose for a lifetime, inasmuch as the 38-year dose from the silos is likewise the total that will be received over a lifetime. If a house has the median background radon level of 1 pCi/L, a person would receive 10-20 WLM in a lifetime (Lubin and others 1995). Using the dose-conversion factor of (20 X 0.65) rems/WLM yields lung doses in the range of 1.3-2.6 Sv. This context allows people to see that the cumulative doses being talked about in the 9 scenarios (0.4-3.4 Sv) are less than what many people naturally receive in their homes. A comparison with indoor radon levels on page S-31would be useful as a way to provide a context for these risks. In addition, the lower bound of the EPA action level of indoor radon is 4 pCi/I, which yields a lifetime lung dose of 5.2-10.4 Sv. It can be seen that the best estimates of cumulative doses from all 9 scenarios are below the ones that EPA has set as the action level.

CONCLUSIONS

It is clear that the Radiation Assessments Corporation has developed a scientific document that can also be used by the Centers for Disease Control and Prevention to determine whether the estimated population doses were sufficient to proceed with an epidemiologic study in the area surrounding the Fernald Feed Materials Production Center. The document contains models and techniques that, although not widely accepted as conventional, show ingenuity in concept and application that might ultimately be important, for example, with respect to decontamination, decommissioning, dose reconstruction, and aerosol physics.

The National Research Council committee believes that the dose-reconstruction approach used provides reasonable estimates of environmental releases of uranium. However, there appears to have been some overestimation of radon releases. Radon is the radionuclide found to be the main contributor to the dose to the lung, the most important organ in this study, so the potential overestimation of the dose is of concern. Assumptions made in estimating risk such as dose-conversion factors and age and sex effects tend, in the committee's view, to overestimate the risk of lung cancer. The overestimates provide the public with information on only the highest possible exposures which would lead to the highest possible risk. Although it is difficult to determine the precise extent of overestimation, it might be by a factor of 4 to 6 and needs to be corrected. The calculations of radon releases, dose conversions, and age and sex weighting factors need to be reevaluated so as to arrive at more-realistic risk estimates.

The project has shown that the most-important combination of source and pathway for radiation exposure is through airborne radon released from the K-65 storage silos, rather than to uranium releases, as was previously believed. Airborne-radon exposures decreased markedly after 1979, the year that the silo vents were sealed; thus, the most-important source of exposure to radioactive materials has now been controlled. Uranium releases to off-site areas account for a smaller contribution to historical dose estimates; this was not previously understood.

The project team has made substantial progress in developing final population dose estimates that could facilitate making decisions on the efficacy of an epidemiologic or health-effects study in the populations living near Fernald. The likely doses that residents around Fernald could have received were developed, with public input, for 9 scenarios that were thought to be generally typical of longer-term, younger residents, although hundreds of scenarios are possible. The dose scenarios are not specific nor do they provide a likely distribution of individual doses; but they might yield an upper-bound estimate for a potential epidemiologic study. The methods developed for these 9 scenarios could also be used to estimate individual doses, but they were not intended to be and were not so applied, because the necessary information for such determinations is expected to be developed in the context of an epidemiologic study. In the final analysis, errors in the input data will add considerable variability to individual risk estimates derived for real, as opposed to hypothetical, people. This should be made clear in the RAC report.

Given the complexity of individual circumstances, not all individuals would fit into any of the selected 9 scenarios. It might be useful to individuals and the community as a whole to make available a questionnaire that could yield more relevant estimates of individual doses. Dose modeling for individuals requires such inputs as date of birth, place(s) of residence and calendar years lived there, locations of schooling and work, dietary habits (percentage of local produce and so on), and amounts and types of outdoor activities. Doses to individuals and the geographic-demographic distributions of residents would permit an estimate of the distribution of doses to the population.

If the results of this dose reconstruction or the data from future dose reconstructions are to be used to determine whether an epidemiologic study should be undertaken, 5 recommendations seem warranted:

- Develop and clearly articulate the objectives of the dose-reconstruction effort. The objectives might include development of dose distributions to evaluate the feasibility of an epidemiologic study, of methods to implement the epidemiologic study, of ranges of potential doses to inform the public, and of individual-dose estimates for the members of the community.

- Obtain community concurrence in the objectives of the study and develop a process for community involvement in their implementation.

- Design an iterative study plan for collecting the dosimetric and epidemiologic data needed to determine feasibility and desirability of proceeding.

- Determine early in the process the kinds of data needed to meet the articulated objectives. The study should be designed to provide all needed data. Resources should be allocated to reduce the uncertainty of the model used. Past efforts tended to evaluate some parameters in considerable detail, whereas others were based on published data that were highly uncertain and of questionable relevance.

- Put into place a study to evaluate and compare past dose-reconstruction efforts. The evaluation might include such issues as whether the desired information was obtained, whether it was presented in the best way (for example, in models at Hanford or exposure scenarios at the Fernald Feed Materials Production Center), and whether public involvement was appropriate.

SPECIFIC COMMENTS ON VOLUME I

The range of cumulative exposures observed in studies of indoor radon exposure is similar to that being discussed here, so an overall, balanced summary of the findings from these studies (including the absolute excess number of lung-cancer cases observed) would be a helpful comparison.

The committee has some additional specific comments:

Page 94, middle paragraph, and table 26: The baseline radiogenic risk of cancer (5%/Sv) that RAC multiplies by 2 for exposures before age 20 years is based on a population of all ages; that is, it includes the population aged 0-19 years. It is more appropriate to multiply by 2 a risk figure for only those aged 20 years and over, which would be 20% lower than what RAC derived.

Page 96: Figure 51, which is reasonable for presenting risk estimates, contains an error. The top left bubble and bracket in the figure incorrectly label the distance from the median to the 95th percentile as the "uncertainty range of additional risk" due to Fernald irradiation. The bracket should instead extend from the 5th percentile to the 95th percentile; the 5th percentile is not even identified on the chart, so there is no place to extend the bracket.

SPECIFIC COMMENTS ON VOLUME II: THE TECHNICAL APPENDIXES

As previously stated, the appendixes to the final Fernald report contain the technical details associated with the dose reconstruction. Because these appendixes are likely to be of interest to others involved in dose-reconstruction projects, the National Research Council committee offers several suggestions.

Appendix H: Particle Size Distributions for Dust Collectors

RAC has chosen to accomplish several things in this appendix, including fitting the cascade-impactor data by exact polynomial equations, simulating mathematically the action of an Andersen impactor by describing the jet configurations and air flows to match the air-sampling process, and comparing this approach to conventional particle-size analysis by using lognormal distribution assumptions and probit analyses to obtain mass median aerodynamic diameters (MMADs). This is an acceptable approach to obtain a more-accurate description of the particles collected on each impactor run, but it is unconventional, and operationally it might be cumbersome or time-consuming.

Several basic statements made in this appendix should be emphasized, as follows.

Page H-2, paragraph 4: "Rather than making the prior assumption that all particle size distributions were lognormal, we fitted cubic polynomials to the log-probability-transformed cumulative sampler data in order to represent the distributions by continuous functions for further calculations. . . . We did not consider possible distortion of the distribution of particles that entered the sampler."

Page H-1, paragraph 6, and page H-2, paragraph 1: "We have examined the properties of the Andersen Mark II cascade impactor, and we have developed a simulation of the instrument to study its potential for distorting the sampled distribution. We have found no reason to alter our approach to representing particle size distributions." This statement indicates that the authors were aware of the "in-field" distortion of particle size distributions that actually occur on sampling, but the theoretical description of the instrument does not indicate such losses, so this theoretical model of the impactor is a proper approach.

Page H-4, paragraph 2: "When we first examined the sampler data from the 1985 NKES study we fitted lognormal distributions to the data as a matter of course, but a critical examination of the plots revealed some cases in which the lognormal distribution was obviously not an appropriate representation of the data (whether the data were properly representative of the distribution taken in by the sampler is a separate question)."

Page H-4, paragraph 3: "Knutson and Lioy (1989) discourage the routine assumption of lognormality for particle size data. The authors are of the opinion that the lognormal distribution has been overused. . . . There are significant departures from lognormality. Such departures are quite obvious in the FMPC cascade-impactor data."

All the above quotations from the text are favorable to the proposed new mathematical approach to analyzing particle-size data as collected by Andersen's cascade impactor. The new approach is considered a scientific breakthrough by the RAC authors, and there is nothing inherently wrong with it. For decades, in fact, the industrial-hygiene field has produced many schemes for describing particle-size data, and this is another acceptable one. The traditional lognormal approach is simple for the field measurements and for a rapid assessment of exposure conditions, and it is likely to continue to be widely used.

A further explanation of this text concerning the new approach is best presented on page H-10, paragraph 3. First, it is known that particles entering an impactor tend to bounce on collection stages and that when this happens, the particles can shatter and be carried on to later stages. They then show up as particles of smaller mass than those which were in the distribution that entered the impactor. The lognormal approach generally eliminates the larger-particle fraction because of this. The authors recognize this when they state that "when particle bounce occurs, distorted efficiency curves are effectively being substituted for the theoretical curves on which the analysis is based." However, little contribution is attributed to this phenomenon, as seen on page H-10, paragraph 4: "In the FMPC sampling, however, we believe the comparisons of the sampling data with the simulated data points, which were computed with the theoretical curves, cast doubt on the presence of such levels of degradation of collection efficiency." This theoretical simulation of the impactor does not account for particle bounce, and the polynomial equations fit the data without accounting for any.

A few statements are perhaps not necessary in the report. For instance, page H-11, paragraph 2 states that "in every case, the simulated data points closely approximate the distribution curve from which they were derived." It would be surprising if they did not. In accepting any problems with the simulation, however, the authors state that "this result reassures us that accepting at face value the sample points from the 1985 NKES study is a reasonable procedure for drawing conclusions about the form of the sampled distribution. It says nothing, of course, about the relationship of the distribution at the time of sampling with comparable distributions over time."

All in all, the computer simulation of the Andersen cascade impactor with the mathematics presented is acceptable. The fact that it is not a conventional approach based on an assumption of lognormality in particle size distributions does not detract from the result. Part of the problem, if there is any, in using such a simulation technique might be related to the fitting of the analytic physical results with the biologic model for deposition and retention after inhalation.

Appendix I: Dosimetric Methods

The following must be borne in mind when combining the above analysis of particle size with the modeling for deposition of particles in various regions of the respiratory tract. Many statements that might be interpreted as matters of opinion by someone applying them to hazard analysis will follow. Some examples are given here.

There is confusion between the authors and the information documented by the Task Group on Lung Dynamics, the basis for the deposition model in ICRP-30 presented on page I-9 in this appendix. For instance, figure I-5 shows the fraction of respiratory tract deposition as a function of MMAD; the results for geometric standard deviations range from 1 to 4.5. We are interested primarily in pulmonary deposition of uranium particles and tracheobronchial deposition of radon progeny. From the figure, using a particle distribution of 2 μm for uranium, deposition in the pulmonary region would vary from about 20% to 30%—a factor of 1.5—in going from a standard deviation of 1 to 4.5. In the smaller particle-size region, such as with radon progeny, the same particle size for absorbed progeny yields deposition of about

5% to 10% in the tracheobronchial region. If the unattached progeny are of concern, a particle diameter of 0.02 μm would yield deposition in the tracheobronchial region of 15% to 25% of that inhaled.

Some statements in appendix I might not be adequately explained:

Page I-10, paragraph 1: "At the expense of accepting this range of variability, it is possible to eliminate the GSD (geometric standard deviation) of the distribution as a parameter." The ranges were discussed immediately above.

Page I-9, paragraph 2: "From these calculations, the Task Group concluded that when the mass median aerodynamic diameter (MMAD) of a distribution is specified, the deposition fraction is relatively insensitive to the GSD of the distribution, within the range of 1.2 and 4.5." It is not clear where this originated, but presumably it was in the original task group report; if so, it is not reinforced by figure I-5 discussed above. It is odd that if a polynomial equation is used to fit the particle-size data, no geometric standard deviations may be derived therefrom, and that it is then concluded that the distribution of the particle size distribution is not important for deposition in the respiratory tract. Perhaps a factor of 1.5 is not important, but it appears to be so in fitting the particle distribution.

Appendix S: Lifetime Risks of Fatal Cancer for Individual Scenarios at the Feed Materials Production Center

Page S-4, table S-2: These risk estimates, which are based on data from the Japanese atomic bomb survivors, are dominated by the digestive tract, with the colon having 17% and the stomach 27% of the total risk. In western populations that have been studied, the percentage of total radiation risk associated with those sites appears to be much smaller. It would have been more appropriate to use risk estimates from western populations. However, given that lung exposure proves to be the main concern in this assessment, this point is minor.

Page S-7: The discussion of risk estimates from uranium-worker studies is inappropriately selective in the data that it emphasizes. In each study, RAC focuses on some subgroup finding with a suggestion of a risk and barely mentions the overall negative findings. For example, regarding the case-control analysis by Cookfair and others (1984), the text focuses on a small subgroup that appeared to show an increased risk (paragraph 2), rather than using the risk estimate for the whole series. Similarly, for the Archer and others (1973) and Waxweiler and others (1983) studies, the text essentially ignores any comparison of the observed deficit in lung cancer with the BEIR IV risk estimate (NRC 1988), but instead focuses on a small apparent excess of lymphohematopoietic cancers in the studies. It should also be noted that the Waxweiler paper includes and updates most, if not all, of the Archer cohort; so there are not 2 independent findings of excess lymphohematopoietic cancers, as the manner of presentation suggests.

Page S-11 and figure S-1: This material is vague in describing risk versus age without specifying whether the age is age at irradiation or attained age at observation. Not until a page later is it made clear that it is age at irradiation.

Pages S-11 and S-12: RAC should provide a table of the adjustment factors for age and sex, so that its calculations could be verified. RAC provides voluminous tables for many other items (such as tables I-1S to I-43S, M-21 and M-22, N-27 to N-31, and R2) but not for these key factors. In addition, figure S-1 for these factors does not show the relative-risk coefficients for ages 0-9 years, although they are obviously important for later calculations.

Table S-14: An explanation of a "truncated normal" distribution would be helpful.

SPECIFIC COMMENTS ON SUMMARY BOOKLET

The committee strongly endorses RAC's effort to inform the public of its findings through the development of a simply written, concise booklet summarizing the radiation doses and risks stemming from past Feed Materials Production Center operations. We find parts of the booklet generally well written, but we take serious exception to the figures on pages 11 and 13, particularly the latter. This figure is misleading. The use of a broken scale distorts the visual impression of the cancer background rate, on the one hand, and the releases from the Fernald facility, on the other. Errors (variation) in background cancer rates are not indicated and there is a desperate need for captions for these figures. Moreover, the scale on the figure on page 13 reads "risk of fatal cancer," seeming to imply any cancer, whereas the report itself rightly emphasizes cancer of the lung, inasmuch as the only potentially important doses are related to radon.

The summary booklet of the report does a poor job of risk communication. This is a complex task for which RAC should have sought more guidance. Nearly all activities that benefit society are also associated with risk. All industrial facilities subject the surrounding community to additional risk (from increased automobile traffic, pollutants, and so on); however, these risks are offset by a variety of benefits. This report estimates the magnitude of the risk associated with the radiologic hazard of this facility but does not compare that risk with the nonradiologic hazards associated with the facility or with other industrial facilities throughout the country. Some concise generic discussion of risks and benefits of industrial facilities would have been helpful.

ADDITIONAL COMMENTS

The radon released to the environment from the K-65 storage silos was found to be the principal pathway for radiation exposure of the surrounding population. The amount of radon released must therefore be estimated with particular care. However, the sections dealing with this in the RAC's task 6 report are not self-contained but rely heavily on information presented in the task 2 and 3 reports and are not reproduced here. Two methods of estimating radon releases are presented, termed the "conventional method" and the "preferred method." These methods are not defined specifically; the closest to a description is shown in a flow diagram (figure 15 in volume I of the RAC report), which does not clearly address the fundamental differences involved.

A better flowsheet for the 2 methods might look like the illustration in figure 1 on the next page. The 2 methods differ essentially in how the original radon source term is obtained. They use the same assumptions regarding escape to the outside air before and after the 1979 sealing of major openings in the silos, and both assume that diurnal warming of the headspace is the principal driving force to radon release.

The Conventional Model

Table Q-1 provides the starting point for this approach. The 2 silos contained roughly 20 million pounds of uranium tailings and process waste with an estimated radium content of 389 mg/ton (with an unspecified assay uncertainty). That translates to a radium inventory of about 389 mg/ton x 10,000 tons = 3,890,000 mg (3,890 Ci of radium), contained in a cylindrical mass about 18 ft high. The waste material consisted mainly of dewatered but moist granular material, so any radon emanation into the headspace would have to come primarily from the top 2 ft of this mass (Zettwoog and others, 1982, Sogaard-Hansen and Damkjaer, 1987). Assuming some homogeneity in the source volume, this layer would contain about 3,890/9 or 432 Ci of radium in equilibrium with 432 Ci of radon.

Table Q-3 lists measured emanation fractions ranging from 0.10 to 0.66; taking a high value of 0.5 results in a headspace inventory—under stable, no-loss conditions—of about 200

Figure 1. A proposed flowsheet to illustrate the fundamental differences between the two methods of estimating radon releases.

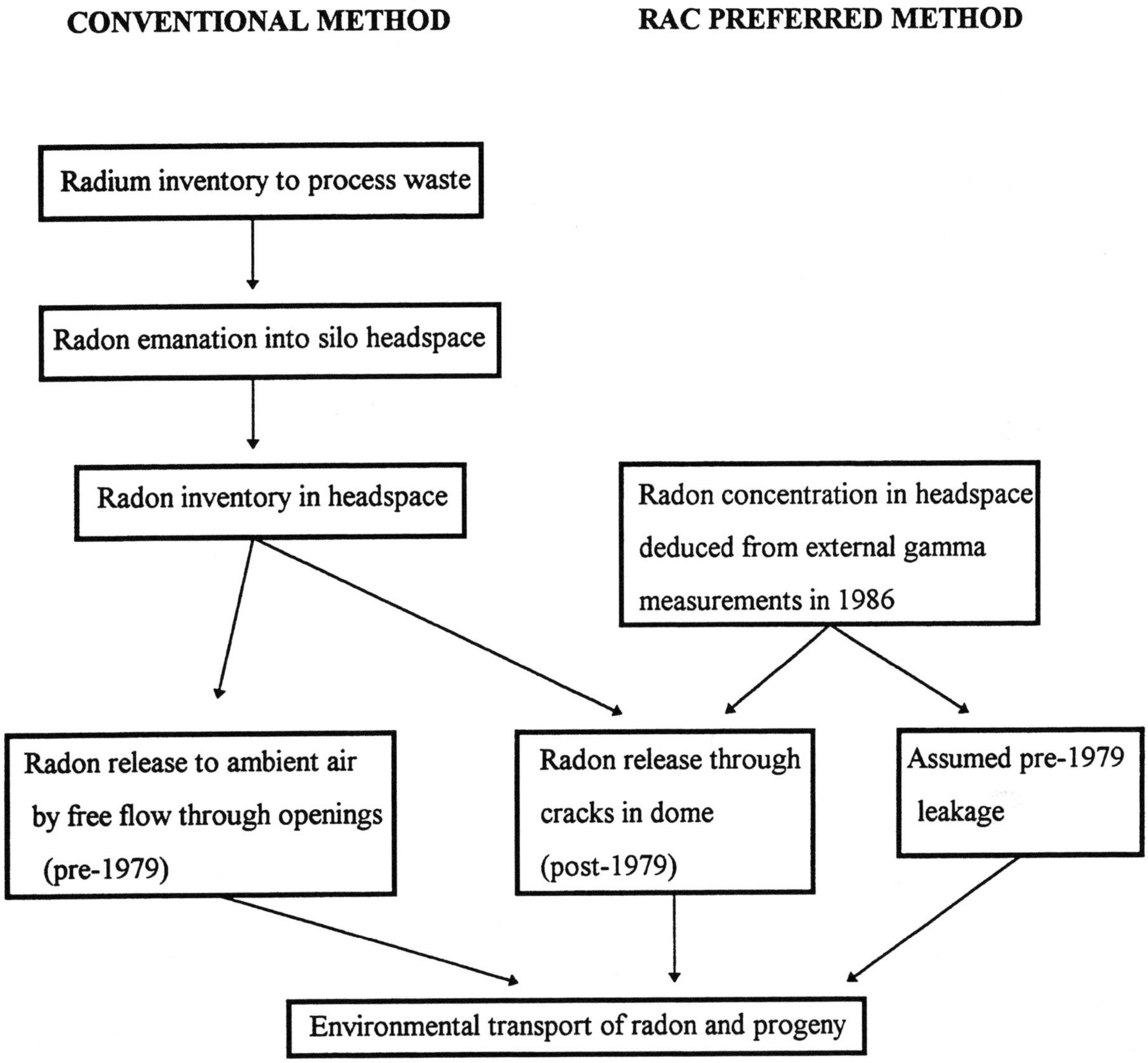

Ci of radon for the 2 silos combined. If the combined headspace volume for the 2 silos is about 57,000 ft^3 (Task Report 2/3, page J-29), this leads to a radon concentration of 3.4 mCi/ft^3, or about 120 μCi/L, assuming minimal outflow. This is a condition that might be encountered after the 1979 "sealing" of the dome.

If one assumes substantial "unconstrained" leakage to the outside under pre-1979 conditions, the concentration would decrease greatly, and the transient concentration in the headspace would be determined by the radon influx from emanation from the waste mass, governed by the 3.68-day half-life of radon-222, and the outflow "leakage" rate via major cracks in the dome. Because there was no obvious entry path to replenish air losses vented to the outside other than inflow through the same cracks during the nightly air-volume contraction, the amount of air and hence the radon lost by diurnal warming are necessarily small; however, actual radon concentrations would be substantially lower than the "steady-state" inventory estimated above. Page Q-12 quotes an earlier Department of Energy estimate of 3,000 pCi/L, equivalent to an effective inventory of about 5 mCi for the 2 silos, perhaps not an unreasonable source term.

The Preferred Method

In his method, the radon inventory was derived from 1986 measurements of the gamma-ray field sensed by a detector held against the outside of the sealed dome. No value is presented for this source term in the task 6 report; reference to page J-41 of the RAC task 2/3 report indicates a 1988 estimate of 26.2 μCi/L ± 100% for the sealed dome, that is, a headspace inventory of 52.8 Ci radon, not an unreasonable fraction of the "steady-state" value of 194 Ci postulated above. Because of the method of determination and the lack of specificity about the timing of the measurement in relation to the dirunal cycle, this value is necessarily subject to a substantial uncertainty. It does, however, agree well with a 1987 measurement of radon concentration (RAC task 2/3 report, page J-28): 22 μCi/L. However, as pointed out above, those values are of little help in estimating releases during the pre-1979 period, when concentrations in the cracked dome were substantially lower, as indicated above, and barely sustained by radon emanation from the waste volume.

Table N-1 lists some measured radon-flux measurements made in 1984 over various locations on the sealed, but cracked silo dome. Flow rates vary substantially with even nominally intact locations competing in some cases with flow at visible cracks. Flow measurements range from 36 to 2.2 X 10^7 pCi $m^{-2}s^{-1}$. A few serious leaks clearly would dominate the outflow. Page N-4 quotes a lower-bound estimate of total radon releases from the 2 silos as 7 X 10^6 pCi/s, corresponding to 2 X 10^{11} pCi for an 8-h daytime release in a volume of 2-6.3 X 10^7 L. This would represent 2-3 headspace volume changes per day—an unlikely scenario, in that it would lead to immediate depletion of the radon in the headspace. The situation would be even more implausible at the pre-1979 leakage rate.

An additional modifying factor might arise from the fact that the silos were downwind of the processing building and therefore subject to a dust plume during the early operating years. That provided a relatively large population of coarser attachment particles which, through close-in gravitational settling, contributed additional radon-progeny depletion of the plume.

REFERENCES

Archer VE, JK Wagoner, and FE Lundin. 1973. Cancer mortality among uranium mill workers. Journal of Occupational Medicine 15:11-14.

Cookfair DL, WL Beck, CM Shy, CC Lushbaugh, and CL Sowder. 1984. Lung cancer among workers at a uranium processing plant. In: Epidemiology applied to health physics. National Technical Information Service, Springfield, VA (U.S. Department of Energy Report CONF-830101). Pp. 398-406.

Dupree EA, JP Watkins, JN Ingle, PW Wallace, CM West, and WG Tankersley. 1995. Uranium dust exposure and lung cancer risk in four uranium processing operations. Epidemiology 6:370-375.

ICRP (International Commission on Radiological Protection). 1988. Limits for intakes of radionuclides by workers. International Commission on Radiological Protection Publication 30. Pergamon Press, Oxford, England.

ICRP (International Commission on Radiological Protection). 1994a. Human respiratory tract model for radiological protection. International Commission on Radiological Protection Publication 66. Elsevier Science Limited, Oxford, England.

ICRP (International Commission on Radiological Protection). 1994b. Protection against radon-222 at home and at work. International Commission on Radiological Protection Publication 65. Pergamon Press, Oxford, England.

Knutson EO, and PJ Lioy. 1989. Measurement and presentation of aerosol size distributions. In: SV Hering, Technical Editor. Air sampling instruments for evaluation of atmospheric contaminants, 7th Edition, American Conference of Governmental Industrial Hygienists. Cincinnati, Ohio, pp. 59-72.

Lubin JH, JD Boice, and JM Samet. 1995. Errors in exposure assessment, statistical power, and the interpretation of residential radon studies. Radiation Research 144:329-341.

NCRP (National Council on Radiation Protection and Measurements). 1984. Exposures from the uranium series with emphasis on radon and its daughters. National Council on Radiation Protection and Measurements Report 77. Bethesda, Maryland.

NRC (National Research Council). 1988. Health risks of radon and other internally deposited alpha-emitters. BEIR IV. National Academy Press, Washington, DC.

NRC (National Research Council). 1991. Comparative dosimetry of radon in mines and homes. National Academy Press, Washington, DC.

NRC (National Research Council). 1992. Report of the committee on an assessment of CDC radiation studies: Dose reconstruction for the Fernald nuclear facility. National Academy Press, Washington, DC.

NRC (National Research Council). 1994. Dose reconstruction for the Fernald nuclear facility—a review of task 4. National Academy Press, Washington, DC.

Rimm EB, E Giovannucci, M Stampfer, G Colditz, L Litin, and W Willett. 1992. Reproducibility and validity of an expanded self-administered semiquantitative food frequency questionnaire among male health professionals. American Journal of Epidemiology 135:1114-1126.

Sogaard-Hansen J, and A Damkjaer. 1987. ^{222}Rn diffusion lengths in soils and sediments. Health Physics 53:455-459.

Stevenson KA, and EP Hardy. 1993. Estimate of excess uranium in surface soil surrounding the Feed Materials Production Center using a requalified data base. Health Physics 65:283-287.

Waxweiler RJ, VE Archer, RJ Roscoe, A Watanable, and M Thun. 1983. Mortality patterns among a retrospective cohort of uranium mill workers. In: Epidemiology applied to health physics. CONF-830101. Health Physics Society, McLean, Virginia, pp. 428-435.

Willett W, L Sampson, M Stampfer, B Rosner, C Bain, J Witschi, C Hennekens, and F Speizer. 1985. Reproducibility and validity of a semiquantitative food frequency questionnaire. American Journal of Epidemiology 122:51-65.

Zettwoog P, N Fourcade, FE Campbell, H Caplan and J Haile. 1982. The radon concentration profile and the flux from a pilot-scale layered tailings pile. Health Physics 43:428-433.